Physiotherapy;
Getting into Physiotherapy, How to Start a Physiotherapy Career,

By

Susan J Santi

Contents

1. What Is Physiotherapy?
2. The History of Physiotherapy
3. Physiotherapy Statistics
4. How to Start a Physiotherapy Career
5. What Are Physiotherapy Costs and Will Insurance Pay?
6. How to Check Physiotherapy Credentials
7. Why Physiotherapy Is So Important in Stroke Rehabilitation
8. How Physiotherapy Can Help With Sports Injuries
9. What Spinal Cord Injury Patients Can Accomplish with Physiotherapy
10. Why Physiotherapy Can Help Women's Health
11. Physiotherapy Helps Postural Problems
12. Pediatric Disorders and Physiotherapy to Help Them
13. Using Physiotherapy to Deal with Occupational Injury
14. The Types of Neurological Conditions and Physiotherapy Used
15. Types of Physiotherapy That Help Lower Back Pain
16. The Busy Field of Geriatric Physiotherapy
17. Why Down Syndrome Physiotherapy Should Be Started Early
18. What Is Chronic Airways Disease and How Can Physiotherapy Help?
19. What Physiotherapy Has to Do with Cardiac Surgery
20. Some Physiotherapy Asthma Management Techniques May Be Questionable
21. The Benefits of Physiotherapy for Amputee Rehabilitation
22. The Alexander Technique of Physiotherapy
23. Conclusion

What Is Physiotherapy?

If you have a muscular-skeletal problem or injury, you might be given a referral to a physiotherapy clinic. If you have gone to one before, you know what to expect. If you are new to this service, you might ask, what is physiotherapy?

Physiotherapy is also known as physical therapy. That answers the question of what is physiotherapy for many people. However, if you have not had any dealings with this form of treatment, you need to know more.

A type of health care, physiotherapy concerns itself with providing physical healing methods for many different kinds of injuries and illnesses. Some of these techniques are done in a hands-on manner, by using massage or manipulation of the muscular-skeletal system. Knowing what is physiotherapy is crucial to getting this kind of help.

Education is a part of what is physiotherapy. A physiotherapist will teach a patient how to care for their injuries. He will teach exercises to do at home so that therapy can continue beyond the walls of the clinic or hospital. He will teach ways to overcome difficulties that cannot be cured.

Another part of what is physiotherapy is rehabilitation. Patients have injuries from sports, car accidents, or assault. These injuries can be treated through physiotherapy. Given the right treatments and an injury that will respond to treatment, much progress can be made. Full functioning may be regained. It may even be possible for them to go back to work rather than being laid up at home.

An answer to what is physiotherapy is what kinds of treatments physiotherapists use. Heat, ice, and ultrasound are used to relieve pain and stiffness. Massage, chiropractic, and other hands-on methods are important. All these methods tend to promote better health, both physical and psychological.

Equipment for helping patients regain their strength and mobility are a part of what is physiotherapy. This equipment may allow a person who is partially paralyzed to get the most exercise possible. This is crucial in maintaining the integrity of their spines and muscles.

What is physiotherapy? It is a carefully planned and executed treatment strategy. It is based upon assessments of the conditions that patients suffer. If all goes well, the patient will return to their original condition. If this is not possible, the goal is for the patient to reach a goal that is the best movement and lack of pain that is possible.

People who are referred to a clinic may ask, what is physiotherapy? However, they will be given quick answers to this question. After an initial evaluation, they will be scheduled for treatments like ultrasound or acupuncture. They will be assigned exercises to do at home. A good physiotherapist will begin treatment right away.

People, who ask what physiotherapy is, often do not consider the preventative side of the field. It is a part of the work of practitioners of physiotherapy to encourage exercises and postures that will help patients avoid physical injuries and conditions requiring their services. An excellent physiotherapist will have fewer return patients, but the flow of people needing physiotherapy continues.

The History of Physiotherapy

At least as early as the days of Hippocrates, massage was used and the history of physiotherapy was begun. The practice of physiotherapy has evolved through the centuries from the earliest forms to the complex system of treatment it is now.

In 460 B.C. Hector was using a type of physiotherapy called hydrotherapy, or water therapy. Professionals use this type of therapy today, although it is more specialized for each type of condition that the patients have.

In 1894, there is the first evidence of a group of nurses in the history of physiotherapy with a Chartered Society. Within twenty years, physiotherapy programs were set up in other countries. New Zealand's started in 1913 and America's in 1914.

The first American professionals in the history of physiotherapy were from the Walter Reed College and Hospital in Portland Oregon. Rather than being called physiotherapists, they were called reconstruction aides. These aides were nurses and they had a physical education background. They were important in the recovery of many World War I veterans.

Research has been done throughout the modern history of physiotherapy. In fact, right near the very beginning, a research study was done in the US. It was published in 1921. Physiotherapy research continues today in a myriad of specialties.

Also in 1921, the Physical Therapy Association was formed by Mary McMillan. This group later became the APTA, arguably the most influential organization in the American history of physiotherapy.

The Georgia Warm Springs Foundation was started in 1924 to deal with the ever-growing epidemic of polio. The foundation offered physiotherapy for these patients. Sister Kinney was known nationally for her work with polio victims. She practiced at the Mayo Clinic. The polio epidemic was a turning point in the history of physiotherapy.

After the polio epidemic had waned, the treatments of choice were massage, exercise, and traction. In about 1950, chiropractic manipulations came on the scene in the history of physiotherapy. This was most common in Great Britain.

After that time, the history of physiotherapy moved from hospitals into other arenas of service. There were, and are, physiotherapists working in clinics, private practices, nursing homes, and schools. The Orthopedics specialty of physiotherapy was born about this time, also.

The International Federation of Orthopaedic Manipulative Therapy came onto the scene, and began making changes and has influenced the profession ever since. Mariano Rocabado was a physiotherapist who had a profound impact. Freddy

Kaltenborn, from Norway, influenced physiotherapy on the east coast of the US. At the same time, Geoffrey Maitland of Australia changed the way training was done in the history of physiotherapy.

The focus during the 1980s history of physiotherapy was on technology. New procedures came about that used computers, ultrasound, electrical stimulation, and other devices. By the 1990s, interest had shifted to manual therapy, with Freddy Kaltenborn again leading the way.

During the history of physiotherapy, training and practice have changed and improved. Many brilliant pioneers have left their marks in the literature and organizations of the field. Physiotherapy is a well-respected profession as a result.

Physiotherapy Statistics

Physiotherapy is a strong force in the field of modern medicine. There have been many new programs started for the study of its practice. Physiotherapy statistics give information about those who practice it and those who benefit from it.

Physiotherapy statistics show that in 2004 there were 155,000 people doing jobs as physiotherapists. That number increases every year. Yet, the number of physiotherapists available is not expected to keep up with the demand. It is said that employment will grow in the field much faster than the average occupation and keep growing until at least 2014.

There were 205 accredited physiotherapy degree programs as of 2004, according to physiotherapy statistics. To be accredited, programs have to offer Master's or doctoral degrees. 111 offered doctoral physiotherapy degrees and the rest offered the Master's.

There are also physiotherapy statistics on where these professionals worked. In 2004, sixty percent of them worked in hospitals or physiotherapy offices. The other forty percent of the jobs were spread out among those that worked in nursing homes, doctor's offices, home health situations, and outpatient centers.

According to the physiotherapy statistics, there are a good many physiotherapists who are in a self-employment status. They contract their services to a variety of clients. Some of these are in homes, but others are in adult day care programs, schools, and any of the other jobs that fall into the forty percent group of where physiotherapists work.

In 2004, physiotherapy statistics show that these professionals earned, on average, around $60,000 per year in salary. Some earned as little as $42,000 per year and others earned as much as $88,000 per year. The highest average salaries earned were in the home health services field, at about $64,000.

In the same year, there is evidence in physiotherapy statistics that most physiotherapists, while working a 40 hour week, worked odd hours to accommodate their patients' schedules. One fourth of physiotherapists only work part-time.

Physiotherapy statistics show a strong use of the services of such professionals by people with lower back pain. 80% of working adults get back pain in their lives to the extent that it hampers their lifestyle. Of all the different reasons a person under the age of 45 would be disabled, back pain is the most common.

It is no wonder that physiotherapy statistics show that these professionals will be needed years from now. The number of people who are developmentally disabled that will reach the age of sixty is said to be set to double in the next dozen years or so. These people will need physiotherapy in order to have a good quality of life.

Physiotherapy statistics show an increased demographic of older Americans today. If you took all the people that are now over the age of 65 and doubled it, you would come up with the number of all the people in history who have ever reached 65.

These physiotherapy statistics point to an ever-growing population of people who will need age-related physiotherapy. If there was ever a time when physiotherapists were needed, it is now and in the years to come.

How to Start a Physiotherapy Career

If one wants to help others with physical problems, one might want to start a physiotherapy career. By doing so, one could learn to evaluate physical problems, create plans for patients, and see to carrying out those plans. A physiotherapy career can be professionally rewarding.

The average physiotherapist is between 25 and 54, earns $50,000 to $60,000, and works in a full-time salaried position. Many of these started out with a BA degree, but the trend is towards hiring MA degree or doctoral degree holders who are beginning a physiotherapy career.

If one is considering a physiotherapy career, the degree one gets in important. A physiotherapy aide can get an entry-level degree at a university, community college, or technical school. This is a two-year degree. After graduation, the physiotherapy aide will perform many jobs in the treatment of patients, under the direction of the physiotherapist.

To begin a physiotherapy career as a professional, one needs to get either a master's degree or a doctoral degree. With the master's degree programs, one may have to enter the program at the same time one starts college. At other places, one simply takes about three years of school after the bachelor's degree. Doctoral degrees have similar requirements.

Before one gets into a physiotherapy degree program, one needs to meet specific requirements. Coursework in various life sciences like biology, anatomy are needed. Also important are courses in fields like psychology and social science.

To choose a school to prepare one for a physiotherapy degree, it is wise to consider whether that school offers clinical experiences as a part of the training. It is also important to be aware of the degrees that are available to earn, and the length of the course of study.

The final step before getting that first job to start a physiotherapy career is accreditation. The Commission on Accreditation in Physical Therapy Education (CAPTE) is tasked with ensuring that physiotherapists are fit for the licensing exam. At that point, the licensure exam must be taken and passed. Employers are impressed with high licensure scores. Once the test is complete, you are ready to start your physiotherapy career.

Once the career is started, there will be several things to consider. One is that many states expect one to get routine updates on one's education. This can be done through workshops and continuing education courses. You will not be able to keep your license without keeping up on the latest knowledge throughout your physiotherapy career.

Also, you may want to consider a specialty. There are physiotherapy career specialties in geriatrics, pediatrics, orthopedics, neurological disorders, and sports medicine, to name a few. By choosing a specialty, you make yourself more valuable, thus earning yourself a higher salary and often more respect. Besides this, you can choose a field that is the most important to you.

You can begin your physiotherapy career by researching schools and finding which ones have the best programs for you. If you do become a physiotherapy professional, you will find both financial and personal rewards await you.

What Are Physiotherapy Costs and Will Insurance Pay?

If you are referred to a physiotherapy clinic for an injury or condition, you might be wondering about the physiotherapy costs. More than that, it is important to find out if insurance will pay for treatment and procedures. These are questions to answer before going to the clinic for help.

The simple answer is that no one can pinpoint the exact amount of treatment a person will need, so overall physiotherapy costs are just an estimate. It is possible for an experienced and skilled physiotherapist to make a fairly accurate approximation of how long treatment will take.

There will usually be a flat clinic or office visit fee. This covers only the basic services of the team. If one does not provide adequate notice of cancellation, a fee can be assessed to recoup the fee that would have been taken in for that time slot. Yet, these are just the beginning of the fees. Physiotherapy costs go far beyond the basic fee.

Physiotherapy costs can vary greatly for different treatment sessions. This is because the same procedures are not always performed. Some cost more than others. To get an accounting of the prices for the different methods used, contact the billing department of the clinic or hospital. There should be a list of each type of treatment.

Since many insurance companies give patients a choice of doctors and physiotherapists, it is wise to discuss fees upfront. Physiotherapy costs may affect you even if you have insurance. This is especially true if your physiotherapist has a preference for many short visits instead of fewer longer ones. This will have a bearing on your deductible.

Then, all one has to do is to keep asking at each session what the next session's procedures will likely be. This way, physiotherapy costs will come as little surprise to one. The only question is what kind of payment arrangements will be made. If the patient has no insurance, all physiotherapy costs will be due in full at the time of service.

Clinics often help arrange the payment of physiotherapy costs by contacting workman's comp or insurance companies for one. This makes it possible for the clinic to collect their fees easily. It also takes the burden of phone calls and paperwork off the patient.

Physiotherapy costs may amount to the price of a deductible and a small co-pay for each visit. The number of visits varies, but there is an average to go on. One or two times a week will usually suffice for four to eight weeks. However, a chronic condition may need much more work.

Physiotherapy costs can be financially crippling, or small change. It depends upon the existence of insurance or the ability of the patient to pay out of pocket. Insurance covers most physiotherapy costs, but if there is any doubt, do not be afraid to ask. Physiotherapy is there to make you feel better, not to make you worry about how much it costs. Anything you can do to keep the focus on recovery will help you.

How to Check Physiotherapy Credentials

When you have physiotherapy done, you are putting your body in the hands of someone you believe to be a trained professional. Pain and disfigurement could result if the procedures are done wrong. That is why it is a good idea to check a therapist's physiotherapy credentials.

Physical therapy aides may play a role in physiotherapy. One is not out of line to ask about what kind of physiotherapy credentials such a person has. The standard may simply be a two-year course of study at a Jr. College or a specialty school. Yet, it is important that the clinic is not just hiring anyone who walks in off the street.

While physical therapy aides can help with certain treatment tasks, it is the physiotherapist that assesses the condition of the patient. This person also plans the course of treatment and specific treatments like special exercises.

This physiotherapist is the person to whom the patient will return for progress reports and who will oversee the work of the physical therapy aide. It is very important to ask for the physiotherapy credentials of this professional.

College coursework beyond the bachelor's degree is required for good physiotherapy credentials. If a physiotherapy candidate meets all the requirements, a master's degree with advanced training will prepare her for work in the field.

Physiotherapy credentials to look for are: Foreign Credentialing Commission on Physical Therapy (FCCPT), International Education

Consultants (IEC), International Consultants of Delaware, Inc. (ICD), International Education Research Foundation (IERF), and International Credentialing Associates, Inc. (ICA). Regardless of whether any of these credentials are required, the CAPTE (Commission on Accreditation for Physical Therapy Education) is the first credential needed.

There are different requirements for physiotherapy credentials in all 50 states. Different physiotherapy credentialing agencies are relied upon in different states. Some require a score of 600 or more on the licensing exam. Some require on-the-job training or professional references from physiotherapists who observe them in training.

Most states also require some ongoing education to keep physiotherapy credentials current. Find out how often the license needs to be renewed in your state. Then, you will know an outdated license when you see one. If you go into a physiotherapist's office and see an old license, ask if that is the newest one. If your physiotherapist is not able to produce a current license, look elsewhere for your physiotherapy.

To check on these physiotherapy credentials, it is possible to contact the state licensing board of physical therapists. One can find the contact information of any state's physiotherapy licensing board online. If all else fails, ask the physiotherapist to provide proof of her own training and licensing. It is to her advantage to encourage trust by being open about her physiotherapy credentials.

There is no need to be suspicious or unfriendly about asking for physiotherapy credentials. Chances are your physiotherapist is perfectly qualified to meet all your needs for physical rehabilitation or help with physical problems. It is important to find out about the physiotherapy credentials, but it is just as important not to make an enemy of your physiotherapist.

Why Physiotherapy Is So Important in Stroke Rehabilitation

Stroke rehabilitation is sometimes an uphill climb. After a stroke, patients can be left with paralysis, especially one-sided paralysis. Pain, as well as sensory deficits, has to be managed. Physiotherapy is a key part of the treatment plan.

Physiotherapists begin stroke rehabilitation very soon after the stroke has occurred, while the patient is still in acute care. The physiotherapist will first do an evaluation to determine what disabilities must be dealt with during stroke rehabilitation.

Some of the possible problems are: lack of strength and endurance, limited range of motion, problems with sensation in the limbs, and troubles walking. Stroke rehabilitation will focus on the problems that the patient displays. A plan for treatment will be devised.

Patients will learn to use limbs that the stroke has made temporarily useless. During stroke rehabilitation, it will be determined whether these limbs will reach their previous potential. If not, the physiotherapist will teach the patients ways to manage without their full use of the limbs.

One problem of stroke rehabilitation is called learned nonuse. This is when stroke patients do everything in their power to avoid using limbs that have been affected by the stroke. If left to their own devices, they will cripple the limb further by letting it atrophy through nonuse.

Physiotherapists use stroke rehabilitation to make sure that patients do indeed work to use their impaired limbs. They can do this in a number of ways. Sometimes it helps for the physiotherapist to tap or stroke the limb they want the patient to use.

If the patient will not easily participate in active range of motion exercises, passive ones can be used where the physiotherapist moves the limb herself. Other times, the patient will try to use the affected limb but will naturally fall back on the limb that is functioning well. In this case, stroke rehabilitation may involve gently restraining the healthy limbs.

It can be a difficult task of stroke rehabilitation to help victims relearn switching from one task to another. This is partly because of problems in the brain. The cues to move the muscles and joints in order to change movements are slow in coming. This is why practice is so important. The more times physiotherapists help a patient with this, the easier it becomes.

Recent studies have revealed that stroke rehabilitation can continue long after the hospital stay. In the past, stroke victims were given a short round of physiotherapy during the time they were in the hospital and for a few weeks shortly afterwards.

New research shows that physiotherapy can promote more advanced stroke rehabilitation if it is continued progressively at home. Patients will learn to walk better. They will gain strength to do daily chores. They will also achieve better posture and more balance, which can prevent falls.

Stroke rehabilitation involves a number of therapies, all designed to restore function to the patient's affected limbs. Electrical stimulation, hydrotherapy, and games have all been used. Stroke rehabilitation is not complete without the help of physiotherapy services.

How Physiotherapy Can Help With Sports Injuries

When players have sports injuries, they turn to physiotherapy for rehabilitation. Physiotherapy, also called physical therapy, offers help whether the player is having surgery to correct the damage or not.

One example of the many sports injuries is an anterior cruciate ligament (ACL) injury. This is an injury to the knee. It is one of the common sports injuries in people who play sports that challenge their knees, such as hockey, skating, skiing, basketball, and of course, football. It can limit the range of a player's motion in that leg, and make the leg weak.

Surgery is sometimes done for these sports injuries, but physiotherapy is always a part of the treatment. The three major exercises done to start the healing process of ACL are heel slides, quad sets, and straight leg raises.

Heel slides are exercises for ACL sports injuries that are easy to understand, but may be painful to do at first. One simply lies on the bed or floor with the foot down. Then, one slides the foot slowly towards the buttocks until it hurts a little, and slides it back. This and the other exercises help prepare the knee for surgery or to heal without it.

Another of the sports injuries that physiotherapy is used for is tennis elbow. One might get tennis elbow from playing tennis, certainly, but it can also come about from any activity that involves twisting the wrist.

Sports injuries like tennis elbow are treated with a comprehensive plan of physiotherapy. Exercises are explained and assigned. Another common procedure for sports injuries is the use of ultrasound. Ultrasound is a way of applying heat deep into the muscle for pain relief.

Electrical stimulation can be used to keep pain from being felt through the nervous system. It is used for tennis elbow and many other sports injuries. Massage and manual therapy can also be used for physiotherapy.

Massage is one of the forms of soft tissue manipulation. However, soft tissue manipulation is to muscles what chiropractic is to bones. It deals not only with muscle, but with tendons and connective tissue as well. It is a specialized field of physiotherapy that has been used for people with sports injuries on many occasions.

As many children's sports teams are becoming ever more competitive, sports injuries among youngsters is increasing. Often, a well-meaning parent will tell the child to shake it off and keep playing. It is even more important for children to get adequate physiotherapy than it is for adults. Children are just developing, and a problem in childhood can lead to lifelong pain.

Some sports injuries happen because something physically traumatic happens to your body. Someone runs into you as you run with the football towards the end zone, for example. Other times, it is simply a matter of the physical demands you put on your body.

Physiotherapy is instrumental in the healing of many sports injuries. Many professional sports teams have physiotherapists on their staffs. In fact, either ACL or tennis elbow can become permanent conditions without the use of physiotherapy procedures.

What Spinal Cord Injury Patients Can Accomplish with Physiotherapy

Sports injuries and car accidents, among other injuries, can cause spinal cord injury. The range of spinal cord injury is wide. Some of these injuries are fairly minor and will heal well with a limited amount of physiotherapy, while others need physiotherapy for the rest of their lives.

As always with physiotherapy, the first step is evaluation. A plan is formulated that will include therapies specific to the kind of spinal cord injury the patient has. Neck injuries can cause quadriplegia, which requires special treatments.

An important issue in spinal cord injury is the level of the damage. If a physiotherapy program is not followed faithfully, the spine will begin to atrophy below the level of the spinal cord injury. The spine will shrink and the whole body below that point will become weaker as time goes by.

It is important that spinal cord injury patients get exercise of some form. They are prone to osteoporosis and heart problems, among other conditions. If there is a total lack of exercise, these risk factors become even more pronounced.

Physiotherapy for spinal cord injury involves exercising and stimulating the nerves and muscles below the level of the damage. This will allow patients with spinal cord injury to stay in good physical condition where they can. That way, if a cure becomes available, they will not be too weakened to benefit from it.

Every exercise the physiotherapy personnel go through with the spinal cord injury patient should be video-taped. This allows work to go on at home with an example of each exercise. Range-of-motion exercises are done by a caregiver, who moves the limbs so that they will not become set in one position.

For spinal cord injury patients who are not quadriplegics, there is physiotherapy using mats. These mats are raised off the floor, and can be operated by a hand crank or a power system. The physiotherapist will give exercises where the patient lies on the side, back, or stomach and works out or sits up and works out.

There are many restorative therapies in physiotherapy for spinal cord injury patients. These include electrical stimulation, biofeedback, vibrational therapy, laser therapy and other stimulation activities. Aqua therapy is also a physiotherapy method that is conducive to progress in spinal cord injury patients.

With all these therapies, spinal cord injury patients can sometimes restore themselves to earlier functioning. Other times, they can simply keep their bodies from deteriorating as they wait for a cure.

Spinal cord injury research is being conducted constantly. Physiotherapy is one of the fields that are being explored. One study is putting spinal cord injury patients in harnesses over treadmills stimulating walking. They are trying to find a way to help people walk again who had given up hope of doing so.

Physiotherapy gives hope for spinal cord injury patients. It allows them to have the most normal functioning that they are currently able to have. Perhaps when a cure comes outcomes will be even better. However, physiotherapy will probably always be needed for spinal cord injury patients.

Why Physiotherapy Can Help Women's Health

The subject of women's health encompasses a range of issues that can be treated by physiotherapy. From pregnancy back pain to incontinence problems faced by older women, physiotherapy is there to help.

Bladder incontinence is a problem for 13 million Americans on any given day. Although some men have this problem, it is present in much greater numbers in the area of women's health.

There are several different kinds of incontinence. Stress incontinence happens when the person coughs or sneezes and urge incontinence means the person has sudden urges to use the restroom, for example. Organ prolapse, such as a tilted uterus, can lead to incontinence, as well as sexual dysfunction. This is another area of women's health physiotherapy can help.

Physiotherapists who work in the field of women's health can correct nearly 70% of incontinence problems. The major exercise used is the Kegel. It is a very specialized exercise, and at least half the people who try to do it on their own fail miserably. It takes biofeedback for many to get it right.

Many of the problems of women's health can be traced to the pelvic floor. The Kegel is the exercise that addresses this part of the anatomy. However, other therapies are used as well. Electrical stimulation is only one of the methods used. Soft tissue manipulation is another treatment that has been tried.

Pelvic pain affects many women's health. It may come from a variety of sources. It can be due to vulvodynia or abdominal surgeries, for example. One can have pelvic pain after falling, especially if one lands on the tailbone. These conditions often curtail sexual activities and lead to an overall deterioration in women's psychological health. Physiotherapy offers many treatments to help these problems.

No discussion of how physiotherapy helps with women's health would be complete without a word about pregnancy. Women who are pregnant know that their bodies go through various changes that can be painful. Low back pain is only one of them.

Physiotherapists can help with this. Gentle exercises can be taught to relieve tension in the back. One is to lie on the floor with the knees up and press the small of the back to the floor. This gives a great feeling of relief. Other exercises strengthen the woman's back, but few people besides physiotherapists know how far to go with exercising when pregnant. Women's health is important at this time, and so is the baby's.

Physiotherapists can also give instructions on what amount of exercise is best for pregnant women. After delivery, physiotherapy is a boon to women's health. It can help get women back into shape and instruct them in taking care of their new child while preventing back problems. Another area of postpartum women's health is the treatment of women who have had cesarean sections.

Physiotherapy can help women's health because there are so many conditions that women suffer. Many of these conditions will respond to physiotherapy. It is only natural that women would turn to a tried and true method for relief.

Physiotherapy Helps Postural Problems

Postural problems have always been a problem; they are even worse in the modern workplace. Too many times people have to reach for their computer mouse, putting them in unnatural positions. There is help for both kinds of postural problems in physiotherapy.

Posture is the way one stands, sits, or walks. It can refer to any normal position that the body usually holds. When the shoulders are hunched forward or the arm is extended in an awkward position, these are postural problems. They can lead to muscle and joint pain, headaches, and other unpleasant symptoms.

Some postural problems are caused because a person has pain in one part of her body. She might count on other muscles to do the work of the ones that hurt. This could lead to an unbalanced or awkward posture. It could cause more pain in the long run.

Postural problems can be treated with physiotherapy such as heat, massage, exercises, and chiropractic manipulation. The first order of business is to reduce the pain. Patients with postural problems usually go in to the doctor with painful symptoms. Heat can be used to ease sore muscles that have been holding the body in unfamiliar poses.

Next, postural problems can be treated by an attempt to reverse the affect the awkward positions have had on the muscles. This can be done by massage. The muscles that are tightened because of poor carriage of the body can be worked until they are less tender.

Some muscles may have contracted, or shortened, due to postural problems. Other muscles which oppose them might have lengthened and weakened. It is necessary to stretch the shortened muscles before trying to strengthen, or tighten, the longer muscles. Physiotherapy exercises have been invented for just this purpose.

Anyone who works with a mouse that is not close enough to their keyboard is prone to postural problems. The first step is to make a better arrangement of the work space. Then, exercises can correct the neck, shoulder, and wrist problems that have resulted from postural problems.

Surgeries, like the Carpal tunnel surgery, are the last resort, as physiotherapy can take care of most of these postural problems before such drastic measures are needed. If one wants to avoid surgery, getting physiotherapy early on is a key. Then, with adequate rearrangement of the workplace, the surgery should never be needed at all.

Chiropractic doctors practice physiotherapy techniques to put the body back into alignment after postural problems occur. They can do manipulations to help the patient regain full range of motion. They can also work on the muscles to ease tension there.

Postural problems are common for people of all ages. They can all find help for these aches and pains. A strict regimen of physiotherapy, along with a restructuring of the work and other environments, can be a positive influence on postural problems. With the right physiotherapist, these patients will be able to sit and stand comfortably again. They will not be defined by their postural problems.

Pediatric Disorders and Physiotherapy to Help Them

It is a sad day when one has to deal with pediatric disorders in the family. Most people believe that children should never suffer from physical problems. Yet, the reality must be faced that pediatric disorders can happen. The good news is that physiotherapy offers some help for them.

Unfortunately, there are numerous pediatric disorders. To name a few, there are: scoliosis, torticollis, Osgood-Schlatter, sports and traumatic injuries, reluctant walkers, developmental disorders, cerebral palsy, and genetic disorders.

Physiotherapy for scoliosis - a curvature of the spine - consists of exercises to strengthen the back. Electrical stimulation is used for this type of pediatric disorders. The stimulation goes directly to the skeletal muscles. Chiropractic is also used in an effort to straighten the spine.

Torticollis is a type of pediatric disorders of the neck. There is a problem with one of the muscles of the neck so that the child is not able to hold his head up straight. The head will be tilted to one side. This chin will jut out on the opposite side of the neck. Physiotherapy can stretch this muscle so that the child can hold his head more normally.

Spinal cord injuries as pediatric disorders are difficult to treat. Children often do not want to do the work that is required to stay ahead of the deterioration that can be caused by this condition. Physiotherapy personnel are challenged to keep the child's spirits up as they teach them how to exercise with and without special equipment.

Brain injuries, including cerebral palsy and strokes are pediatric disorders that must be managed delicately. The neurological system is often not as sturdy as the skeletal or muscular systems. However, brain injuries also involve these other systems as well.

A new treatment for these pediatric disorders like brain injuries is using hyperbaric oxygen therapy. This type of physiotherapy is based on the idea that, in these conditions, there are often parts of the brain that are not working but can be revived. The HBOT can sometimes revive them.

Pediatric disorders such as sports injuries and traumatic injuries require different types of physiotherapy based upon the location and severity of the injury. If a child has repeatedly sprained the same ankle, therapy will necessarily focus on that ankle, as well as any body part that supports or counterbalances that ankle. Overall strength is important.

Traumatic injuries require a certain amount of psychological training, as the subject of the accident or other ordeal may bring on such distress that the child does not want to work. A good physiotherapist will be able to work with such a child. Traumatic injuries can also be severe enough that the physiotherapist plans a lengthy course of therapy to overcome them. Pediatric disorders like this require patience from everyone involved.

The list of pediatric disorders is long and varied. Not all of them can be helped by physiotherapy at this time. Right now, physiotherapy can be used in many cases to relieve symptoms or even to reverse damage. Physiotherapy performs a valuable function in helping children live more normal lives.

Using Physiotherapy to Deal with Occupational Injury

There is less occupational injury going on in the last few years than before. This is partly because of the influence of physiotherapy on the workplace. Physiotherapy principles are being used to design better work places and work habits. They are also important in dealing with the occupational injury that does happen.

Occupational injury problems include back and neck problems, carpal tunnel syndrome, shoulder and knee dislocations, tennis elbow, and leg and ankle strains. Physiotherapy can be used to treat any of these conditions.

Back and neck problems are major examples of occupational injury. They happen because of improper lifting, lifting while turning, repetitive turning, or sitting improperly. Workman's comp will probably take care of treatment if the occupational injury is more than a slight one.

Carpal tunnel syndrome is often seen in offices. However, it may also occur in other jobs, such as on assembly lines. Tennis elbow can be an occupational injury as well, occurring any time one repetitively twists one's wrists. This movement is often done in packing plants, for example, as workers twist products into containers.

Patients who have an occupational injury are often put on light duty. Some are even laid off. Physiotherapists can step in and help the patients recover their strength and health. Physiotherapy techniques may include exercises, massage, and ultrasound.

A physiotherapist will certainly give instructions about how to do home treatment. When the occupational injury is sufficiently healed, the patient will be given the go-ahead to return to work. If the patient was on light duty, he will be told when to go back to regular duty. If he was off work, he will be told when he can go onto light duty, and then the full daily routine.

Physiotherapy ideas can also be used to construct a better work environment. The work station in an office can be set up to accommodate the proper positioning of the body. This will ward off occupational injury caused by repetitive movements, like carpal tunnel syndrome.

Occupational injury caused by awkward movements in the workplace can also be eliminated if the work environment is set up in an ergonomic fashion. Physiotherapists have much knowledge about the way the workplace should be constructed.

Physiotherapists know what equipment is best used to avoid occupational injury. Ergonomic keyboards are recommended and correct mouse placement is crucial. The physiotherapist will suggest that you use a touch pad instead of a mouse if at all possible.

Physiotherapists can be very helpful in preventing occupational injury in any other type of workplace. They may be called in to consult with employers and ergonomics specialists about what changes need to be made to make the work environment acceptable for their patients.

Work environments are safer than they once were. Ergonomics principles are used and in many cases are required by law to be used if requested by workers. Workers who are injured have good physiotherapy available to them. However, until there is no occupational injury, physiotherapy will continue to have value in the workplace.

The Types of Neurological Conditions and Physiotherapy Used

Neurological conditions may be very severe. They can be life-threatening at times, and they can certainly affect the quality of the patient's life. There are many neurological conditions and physiotherapy can help many of them.

Alzheimer's disease takes away the declining years of many older people. It is surprising to note that it can occur in people 40 years old or younger. ALS or Lou Gehrig's disease is a disease that robs the brain and spinal cord of the ability to move. Both of these are neurological diseases that can be helped by physiotherapy.

MS, another of the neurological conditions that affects the brain and spinal cord, can lead to a long, slow decline. Parkinson's disease is another of the neurological conditions of the brain. This one can cause shaking and loss of coordination, and problems moving and walking. Physiotherapy offers some relief to these patients.

Guillain Barre Syndrome is one of the types of neurological conditions that affect the brain and spinal cord too. It is a case of the person's own immune system attacking outside these areas. It can be severe enough to require emergency hospitalization. Physiotherapy offers help with regaining strength and adapting to life with the disease.

Neurological conditions that are autoimmune diseases are difficult to treat. Myasthenia Gravis is one such illness. It causes muscular weakness because of a lack of communication between nerves and muscles. Like other neurological conditions, it can be very debilitating.

A great amount of physiotherapy is needed to help Myasthenia Gravis patients to live with their neurological conditions. This includes strength training, training in the use of supportive devices, and help with common tasks. One problem physiotherapist's face when working with MG patients is that too much exercise will make their condition worse and not better.

Many of the patients with neurological conditions cannot carry on daily functions such as caring for themselves and their homes. It is not uncommon for these people to be unable to work. They may even have trouble walking or getting up and down stairs at all.

Difficulty swallowing or breathing; dizziness, poor balance and falls, and a total lack of endurance plague many of these patients who have neurological conditions. Medications or surgeries can help with some of their problems, but many problems are ones they will have to abide. Physiotherapy can offer solutions that other branches of medicine cannot.

Exercises, as in most physiotherapy, include strengthening and stretching exercises. In whatever way is possible, patients with neurological conditions need to get aerobic exercise. Physiotherapists may be able to make a plan so that this is possible.

Part of this plan for patients with neurological conditions would include balance training and coordination training. With these two skills in place, the patient will have a more advanced ability to do aerobic and other exercises. Aquatic exercise is also used.

Patients with neurological conditions must live with many problems of lack of movement and function. Physiotherapy can help them to overcome some of these problems. It can make their lives easier and more pleasant, besides.

Types of Physiotherapy That Help Lower Back Pain

Lower back pain plagues Americans to the extent that 80% will suffer from it at some time in their lives. It is one of the most common reasons people visit the doctor. For many, the problem is more than a passing incident; they need physiotherapy.

Physiotherapy of different types can be used to treat lower back pain. Acupuncture is fast becoming an important method for the relief of such pain. The doctor has the patient lie face-down and inserts the acupuncture needles across the back. The doctor then finishes the procedure for lower back pain. Pain relief after a series of treatments usually lasts months.

Massage is also used for lower back pain. The massage used must be done by someone well-versed in the treatment of lower back pain. A massage done by an untrained person may do more harm than good.

These methods are called passive therapies, or modalities. They are done to the patient and not by the patient. There are other modalities that are commonly used. Heat and ice packs are a well-known form of passive physiotherapy. They can be used separately, or they can be used alternately by a person who is suffering from acute lower back pain.

A transcutaneous electrical nerve stimulator (TENS) can be used as another modality for lower back pain. The patient will feel the sensation of the stimulator instead of his pain. If the TENS unit seems to work well for him, he will be sent home with one to use at his convenience.

Ultrasound is especially useful as a passive therapy for anyone with acute lower back pain. It delivers heat deep into the muscles of the lower back. This not only relieves pain. It can also speed healing.

Back exercises may be assigned by a physiotherapist. These exercises will help with lower back pain if one does them correctly and faithfully. The only exception is if the back is in an acute condition requiring emergency care or surgery.

The exercises that will help with lower back pain the most will be assigned and supervised by a physiotherapist. They may be done at home, but it will be necessary to follow instructions and check in frequently.

These exercises include ones for lower back pain that stretch or extend the back and ones that strengthen it. One is an exercise where one lies prone and moves as if swimming. This protects the back while giving the surrounding muscles a workout.

Lower back pain exercises called flexion exercises strengthen the midsection to provide support for the back. If the lower back pain is reduced when one sits, these exercises are important. One is a knee-to-chest exercise.

Aerobic exercise such as walking is excellent for reducing and preventing lower back pain as well. Massage and acupuncture can be counted on to relieve pain for most patients. Exercises can make the back stronger to both relieve and prevent lower back pain. Any physiotherapy that can help relieve lower back pain will help millions of people.

The Busy Field of Geriatric Physiotherapy

Clinics that specialize in geriatric physiotherapy never run low on work. The elderly have diseases and disorders in greater numbers than any other age group. Their care is difficult, but rewarding.

Geriatric physiotherapy became a specialty of physical therapy study in 1989. Since then, physiotherapists have worked to understand the problems of the aging. There is a long list of problems dealt with in geriatric physiotherapy.

Alzheimer's, arthritis, balance disorders, cancer, cardiovascular disease, incontinence, joint replacement, pulmonary disease, stroke, and osteoporosis are only a few of the problems covered by geriatric physiotherapy. Physiotherapists have a whole range of therapies for these ailments.

The types of problems faced in geriatric physiotherapy are grouped into three different categories. One category is the problems that happen because the patient simply does not use their limbs or does not exercise. These problems can be addressed by reconditioning through range-of-motion exercises and other exercises.

Another category geriatric physiotherapy deals with is cardiovascular disease, like heart disease and stroke. The physiotherapy professional has an array of tools at her disposal to work with these conditions. Exercise, aqua therapy, electrical stimulation, and more can be used.

The third category is skeletal problems. Geriatric physiotherapy helps people who have these disorders, such as osteoporosis and osteoarthritis. These problems require special attention as osteoporosis makes patients frailer, and osteoarthritis is very painful.

Because falls are such a problem, the osteoporosis therapy is crucial. Along with that, geriatric physiotherapy is responsible for preventing many falls because of work with balance and gait. Some clinics focus entirely on balance issues for the elderly.

Much of the work of geriatric physiotherapy is not aimed at returning patients to their earlier states of health. The most important goals are to be able to function at their best abilities. Doing everyday tasks and living an unconfined life are valuable assets.

At the same time, geriatric physiotherapy can have a profound affect on a person's ability to enjoy physical activities. Golf is an activity that many seniors enjoy. It can be a very hazardous sport for the elderly if they are not in condition to play. It does have many health benefits, too.

Geriatric physiotherapy can focus on physical training to get an older adult in shape to play sports like golf. This strengthens them in many ways. The fact that it allows them to play golf will make them even healthier, both physically and psychologically. Since depression is a growing problem among the elderly, any help they can get in this area is needed.

Another role of geriatric physiotherapy is to help with rehabilitation after knee or hip replacement surgeries. People who have these operations are likely to walk differently. It affects their abilities to do daily chores, and their quality of life. Physiotherapists can help.

Some people turn to physiotherapy as a means of better functioning. Others are referred to physiotherapy clinics by their doctors for specific problems. Still others end up in geriatric physiotherapy care in hospitals or nursing homes after accidents or illnesses. All of these people can be helped.

Why Down Syndrome Physiotherapy Should Be Started Early

There is a great need for immediate intervention for children with Down syndrome. Physiotherapy does not fix the problem; development will still be slowed. However, it can address problems that are unique to Down syndrome children.

Early Down syndrome physiotherapy focuses on four problems that are common for these children. One is called hypotonia. This means that the child's muscles lack tone. That is why, when you lay a Down syndrome child in his crib, he will flop out like a rag doll. Hypotonia needs to be treated because it affects the ability of the child to learn motor skills or to support himself correctly.

Another problem that can be helped by Down syndrome physiotherapy is laxity of the ligaments. The ligaments are so loose that they do not support the bones adequately. In infancy, it can be seen in the way they lie down with their legs splayed apart. In later years, their ankles and other joints will be loose enough to cause support problems.

Down syndrome physiotherapy is essential in helping these children overcome muscular weakness. If they are not exercised to correct the problem, they will develop behaviors that will make up for their lack of strength. Some of these behaviors may be harmful. For example, they may lock their knees to make up for having weak legs.

One problem these children face is in their body shape. Their arms and legs are generally shorter compared to their trunks than in most people. This leads to all kinds of problems sitting and climbing. Just reaching the table to eat can be a chore. Down syndrome physiotherapy can help with this problem.

In early intervention Down syndrome physiotherapy, the emphasis is on overcoming weakness and learning gross motor skills. Rolling over, sitting, crawling, and walking will all happen eventually, anyway. However, with Down syndrome physiotherapy, they can take place with solid physical foundations.

There is a concern with Down syndrome physiotherapy of parents notifying the doctors of problems that might require the help of a physiotherapist. A parent may be at a loss as to what is to be considered worthy of attention. After all, they already know that their child is not like other children who do not have Down syndrome.

If parents see a Down syndrome child having trouble holding up her neck, it is essential to call it to the attention of the doctor so that physiotherapy can be ordered to strengthen neck muscles. This is one example of many where a physiotherapist might help.

Once Down syndrome physiotherapy is started, it is best to keep up a life-long program to maintain health. Prevention of age-related problems with bones, ligaments, and muscles is becoming increasingly important. This is because people with Down syndrome are living to older ages. In fact there are more Down syndrome people over the age of 60 than ever before. Physiotherapy can help them live quality lives.

Down syndrome physiotherapy is often ignored until much damage has been done. The children are left with weaknesses, odd behaviors, and disfigurements that need not have happened.

If Down syndrome physiotherapy is started early enough, the child will have a much healthier life.

What Is Chronic Airways Disease and How Can Physiotherapy Help?

Chronic airways disease is actually a group of diseases. These diseases are also called chronic obstructive pulmonary disease (COPD). Chronic airways disease can cause a major change in the quality of a patient's life. However, physiotherapy can help.

Diseases included in chronic airways disease are chronic bronchitis and emphysema, for example. Many other diseases that restrict or limit breathing are included. It is most often caused by cigarette smoking, but also can be caused by inhaling other irritants such as those in the workplace. Chronic airways disease is more common among the elderly.

Along with having shortness of breath, the patient is likely to wheeze and cough frequently. He will produce sputum in copious amounts, and sometimes that will be streaked with blood. The lips and fingers can take on a bluish tint because he is not getting enough oxygen, and heart trouble may follow for the same reason.

Physiotherapy can help with chronic airways disease in many ways. One is in breathing retraining. This is just what it sounds like. A physiotherapist works with the patient to teach him ways to breathe that will draw the most air while eliminating the most wheezing. This can be a great help for those with chronic airways disease.

Another method used by physiotherapists for those with chronic airways disease is called clapping and postural drainage. The postural drainage part is done by positioning the body so that the affected lung is above the trachea.

Many people do this at home by lying on a bed and bending the top half of the body over it. The physiotherapist teaches one how to do this so that the lung will drain. Before long, the patient with chronic airways disease will be doing this procedure on his own.

The other part of the help for chronic airways disease patients is called clapping. This is done by cupping the hand and clapping the back to loosen secretions in the chest. It is also called chest percussion. The physiotherapist will do this procedure, and will teach it to a family member or caregiver.

People with chronic airways disease often have a problem with weakening legs. This is because, as they have trouble breathing, they avoid walking or doing physical exercise of any sort. The goal of physiotherapy in this case is to strengthen the legs through treadmill-walking or stationary-cycling. This can only be done, however, if the patient is well enough to start out.

Conditioning the arms of chronic airways disease patients is just as important. Most daily jobs rely heavily on the arms to do the work. Exercises which focus on the arms not only strengthen the muscles of the arms. They also help the patient start breathing better.

Chronic airways disease is a condition that can benefit from physiotherapy. The physiotherapist treating the patient must have specialized knowledge for this type of treatment. Simple methods can be overlooked as modern treatments come to the forefront. Yet, physiotherapy personnel who know this technique can make a big difference in patients' lives.

What Physiotherapy Has to Do with Cardiac Surgery

One may feel fatigued and sore after cardiac surgery; it is only natural. On the other hand, it seems altogether strange to think of embarking on a course of physiotherapy afterwards instead of just resting. Yet, that is just what is recommended.

Types of cardiac surgery include bypass surgeries, angioplasty, stents, heart valve replacements, and even heart transplants. Patients having all of these surgeries can benefit from physiotherapy. Patients who have other cardiac problems can use the help too; they include victims of heart attacks, heart failure, peripheral artery disease, chest pain, and cardiomyopathy.

Physiotherapy will usually begin within a couple of weeks of cardiac surgery, if not sooner. The first step is for nurses or doctors to administer a stress test to determine how much exercise one can handle. This involves walking on a treadmill or riding on a stationary bike while having one's vital signs monitored.

When the data is gathered and analyzed, a program of physical therapy will be put into place. For safety's sake, it is often the routine to bring cardiac surgery patients into the hospital or an outpatient clinic for their exercise at first.

Under the watchful eyes of nurses and physiotherapy personnel, cardiac surgery patients will be looked after as they perform their exercises. This way the professionals will be alerted if the cardiac surgery patient is having troublesome symptoms. The exercises done are cardiovascular exercises like walking on a treadmill or riding a stationary bike.

After the initial period of the monitored physiotherapy has passed, cardiac surgery patients will be sent to do their exercising at home. Before they go, though, they will have been taught warm-up and stretching exercises, and when to stop. Generally, they should exercise three to five times a week unless they are having problems.

Swimming is another form of exercise that is especially good for cardiac surgery patients. It is a cardiovascular exercise that is not hard on the joints, so it will often be kept up longer. The only thing to remember is that all wounds must be completely healed first.

Physiotherapy for cardiac surgery patients is often not carried out by physiotherapy staff. Nurses in hospitals and clinics who are trained to deal with these areas of rehabilitation for cardiac surgery will do the work. However, physiotherapists sometimes help, and the principles are the same.

The physiotherapist will instruct the patient about what activities are acceptable in the weeks and months after surgery. During the first six weeks, there will only be a few activities allowed, such as light housekeeping or going to movies, for example. From then until the third month, more activities will be added. You may be able to return to work, at least part-time, you may be able to drive. After this time, your physiotherapist will work with you to ease you back into all your old activities.

If a patient has cardiac surgery and then does nothing to regain strength, that patient will soon weaken. Physiotherapy offers a means to stay in shape, or get into shape. It lends more purpose to the cardiac surgery by making the patient much healthier than before the surgery ever took place.

Some Physiotherapy Asthma Management Techniques May Be Questionable

Physiotherapy Asthma management is a concern for about 15 million people in America. There are many different medications and other treatments used successfully for asthma management. However, some methods used are not quite proven to work.

Some physiotherapy clinics claim that massage can be used for asthma management. They state that it works to relieve the symptoms of wheezing and breathlessness. They use massage on patients young and old. However, there is no substantial proof that massage does any more good for asthma management than to relieve stress.

One alternative physiotherapy method that has been used for asthma management is acupuncture. There is some indication that this technique can actually have some benefit in relieving symptoms of asthma.

Acupuncture does seem to help the immune system fight off illnesses. This is important in helping asthma management. Illnesses such as colds or flu will exacerbate the asthma condition. If acupuncture can reduce this, it is a great help. Yet, acupuncture is still only recommended to be used along with other treatments. It is not to be used alone.

Some acupuncturists use other methods for asthma management. They might burn herbs over acupuncture points. They might give patients a certain kind of massage, or teach them breathing exercises. There is no known validity in these treatments.

Chiropractors rely on spinal manipulation for asthma management. The reviews of this theory are mixed. One study compared a sham, or fake, type of spinal manipulation that was done on one group of asthma patients. The other group got the real manipulations. There was little, if any, difference between the two groups. This would suggest that chiropractic adjustments are not effective for asthma management.

However, another study was done. Eighty-one children were followed through asthma management at a chiropractic clinic over a period of time. Overall, there were 45% fewer asthma attacks among these children after treatment. 30% were able to significantly reduce their asthma medications. Thus, the jury is still out on the effect of chiropractic medicine on asthma management.

There is a physiotherapy specialty certification for those who wish to work with asthma management. Physiotherapists may take a test to become certified as Certified Asthma Educators, and they help people to deal with their condition. What is more, Medicare and Medicaid pay for their services.

There is also some evidence that asthma management for those who have to be admitted to the hospital should involve physiotherapy. There was a study of respiratory patients who were given range of motion exercises while in the hospital. The average stay was three days less than those without the exercises.

One challenge of traditional physiotherapy for asthma management is that dehydration happens easily. Asthmatics get dehydrated more easily, and it affects them in a worse way. It can even bring on an asthma attack. Any exercise plan must take this into account.

There are ways for physiotherapy to be used for asthma management. Certainly, there are other methods, and research may prove these methods have value. In the meantime, some methods are better saved for alternative methods to be used in addition to medications and proven physiotherapy treatments.

The Benefits of Physiotherapy for Amputee Rehabilitation

Losing a limb is a devastating blow for anyone. It requires a team of professionals to make the adjustment to life without the limb. A physician, a prosthetist, nurses, and a psychologist are all needed. Add to that list a physiotherapy service, which will help with amputee rehabilitation.

The benefits of physiotherapy for amputee rehabilitation are numerous. For one, amputees will need help in overcoming phantom pains. These are pains where the limb used to be. The sensation really is in the nerve that would lead to that limb if it were still there. Physiotherapy can use its own techniques to treat this pain.

Most amputees will be getting a prosthetic limb. Some feel that it should be enough to learn how to put it on. It is not an automatic thing to get used to a prosthetic limb. Many patients have them for years without ever having normal functioning with them. This is one reason amputee rehabilitation is so important.

Physiotherapy can benefit amputee rehabilitation by gradually getting the patient accustomed to using a prosthetic limb. The physiotherapy plan for this will be based upon the needs and abilities of the patient.

The patient will probably need help during amputee rehabilitation to learn balance all over again. This is especially true is the affected limb is a foot or leg. However, having an arm that is of a different weight than the other may be unbalancing as well. Physiotherapy can help with these problems too.

One thing people going through amputee rehabilitation need to realize is that gait is a good deal of the battle. If one walks correctly, people will not even be able to detect one's limp, even with a prosthetic leg. This skill can be learned from physiotherapists.

If a patient has waited a long while before seeking physiotherapy after surgery, a problem may arise. Certain muscles may become overdeveloped and others weakened. This happens because, without proper amputee rehabilitation, the patient relies on one set of muscles to the exclusion of others. A proper plan of physiotherapy can address this issue.

People who have lost a limb will need an individualized exercise program. Physiotherapy can provide such a program during amputee rehabilitation. This will take into account the different movements needed by amputees to perform normal exercises.

Manual therapies, such as massage, are a part of amputee rehabilitation with physiotherapy. This can relieve much pain and tension in the muscles that are overworked in getting used to their new situation. Other treatments can be used. Some of them are heat, acupuncture, ultrasound, and electrical stimulation.

There is a need for physiotherapy in amputee rehabilitation that no other discipline can fill. It is a basic kind of help that anyone who has lost a limb can use. Some amputees decline treatment because they do not think it is necessary. Others feel overwhelmed by their loss. If there is a way to convince amputees to get physiotherapy to help them with their rehabilitation, they will find recovery a much smoother path.

The Alexander Technique of Physiotherapy

The Alexander Technique was invented by a man named F.M. Alexander. He lived from 1869-1955. He was an actor, touring Tasmania and Australia with a Shakespearean troupe. He began to have problems with his voice, and the rest is history.

When Alexander's throat became extremely hoarse, he made the rounds of all the doctors where he was at any given time. None of them could help him. They could not find any physical reason for the problem. The Alexander Technique came about because the man would not take no for an answer.

Since there was no one to come to his aid, Alexander began watching his every move. He spent much time looking into mirrors, trying to determine what he might be doing wrong. Over a period of nine years, he came up with a solution: the Alexander Technique.

The system Alexander designed did the trick of restoring his voice. This was nothing short of a miracle for him. His voice was of utmost importance to him as an actor. He did not name the system the Alexander Technique, though. He named it primary control.

The hypothesis of the Alexander Technique is that the head, neck, and torso are the primary factors in determining function, movement, and posture. In other words, these body parts control these features of the human anatomy.

Through his observations, he learned that by compressing these body parts, the body did not work in accordance with its design.

In his case, this led to poor posture, which resulted in the hoarseness of his voice. For others, he saw that there were other problems that the Alexander Technique, or primary control, could help.

Primary control, as Alexander used it was the correct positioning of the head, neck, and torso so that the body worked normally. Now, the Alexander Technique is being used in clinics around the country. It is taught to people who are young and people who are old. It is taught to anyone comes to be taught.

Alexander Technique practitioners usually work with people on an individual basis. Groups can sometimes be taught the Alexander Technique, but this is not standard practice. The key is for the practitioner to employ physiotherapy techniques and education to help the person to use their body better and function better overall.

The idea of the Alexander Technique is to provide a physiotherapy that will allow muscles to become relaxed. This is said to give people back the posture they should have had all along. The body is worked with the human form as a whole, and so doing the Alexander Technique is said to have effects for all parts of the body.

The Alexander Technique is a highly specialized area of physiotherapy. This technique addresses issues that are related to posture only, albeit there are many problems that are. It is generally not used for people with major disabilities or illnesses. Other forms of physiotherapy are better for those patients. However, for people with minor problems, the Alexander Technique has been known to work wonders.

Conclusion

So here we are at the end of my book; Physiotherapy. This is a truly wonderful profession and one of the most rewarding. To see someone transform with your guidance is very special.

It is also a profession in which you will grow and discover things about yourself. It's a lifelong journey.

Finally please leave a review as they really help me continue to do this and put of informative ebooks on this subject.

All the best

Susan

Printed in Great Britain
by Amazon